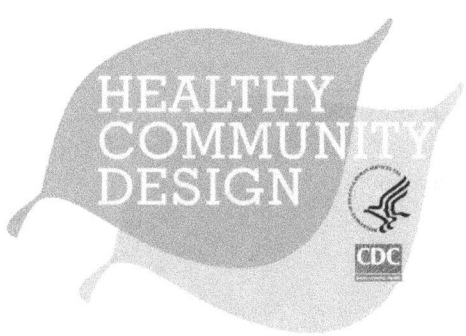

# Healthy Community Design Expert Workshop Report

September 21-22, 2009
Centers for Disease Control and Prevention
Atlanta, Georgia

# Table of Contents

VII.   Tool for evaluating objectively the potential health effects of a project or policy before it is built or implemented: Health Impact Assessments (HIA)

    a.   Definition

    b.   State of the HIA

    c.   Real and perceived barriers


VIII.  The path forward

    a.   Summarize ideas for CDC initiatives

    b.   The contributions industry groups can make


IX.    Conclusion

    a.   Summarize participant evaluations

    b.   Keeping the conversation going

# I.    EXECUTIVE SUMMARY

On September 21 and 22, 2009, the Centers for Disease Control and Prevention (CDC) convened a group of 20 experts in the field of community design to discuss raising awareness about the health impact of community design decisions. The gathering included top thought leaders whose organizations represent those who play a direct role in creating the built environment through action and policy—developers, architects, planners, builders, academia, public health professionals, and government officials. Its interdisciplinary nature was both unique and intentional.

The workshop was conceived as a result of a series of interviews in September and October 2008 that CDC had conducted with professionals in the public health, planning, and built environment sectors. From these interviews, two key themes emerged:

- A common concern about health exists, but common language among the disciplines is lacking.
- Almost no cross-discipline synergy on shared health concerns exists, and local public health professionals are not in the loop at the critical early stages of policy and project development.

Interviewees agreed that CDC, as one of the leading national authorities on public health issues, has the credibility to convene the conversation on these issues. The Healthy Community Design Expert Workshop was conceived as a result of interview feedback.

The desired outcome of the Healthy Community Design Expert Workshop was for participants collaboratively to develop action steps to expand awareness of the health impact of community design decisions. CDC also hoped that the workshop would result in future collaboration among participants in promoting and conducting research on healthy community design.

In the long term, CDC hopes that the strategies developed from this workshop will lead to the

(1) Inclusion of public health impact in the training of built environment professionals;

(2) Recognition by public health professionals that collaborating with architects, planners, transportation planners, and developers is key to advancing healthy community design;

(3) Consistent promotion and publication of best practices; and

(4) Objective evaluation of potential health effects of a project or policy by all relevant parties *before* it is built or implemented.

To create context for the conversation, all participants were asked to share healthy community design best practices or effective policies. Participants then chose five of the practices or policies for break-out group discussions on how to encourage their widespread adoption. Projects discussed included Miami-Dade, Florida; Garland, Texas; Lakewood, Colorado; Tysons Corner, Virginia; and Decatur, Georgia.

Ideas that came out of the break-out group exercise fell under the following categories:

- Research: Market to community design influencers scientific research, anecdotes, and case studies that show the health benefits of considering the health impact of design in projects and policies before they are built or implemented

- Leadership/Ownership: Identify champions and tag teams to see projects through

- Messaging/Communications/Marketing: Establish a healthy community design movement among influencers who can have the most positive health impact on the built environment, focus the discussion on establishing a standard practice among influencers that considers the health impact of a project or policy before it is built or implemented

- Financials: Reconsider the tax base, offer incentives, identify funding sources

- Strategy: Aim for scalability, consider demographics, encourage mixed land use and greater land density among urban planners and developers; revise zoning laws to allow mixed use

Participants discussed the Health Impact Assessment (HIA) as one of the tools currently available to facilitate communication and partnerships between health professionals and decision-makers in the built environment. A representative from Health Impact Project (a collaboration of the Robert Wood Johnson Foundation and Pew Charitable Trusts) was on hand to announce the new HIA grant funding program that will also provide technical assistance to grantees. Participants shared the following concerns about HIAs:

- What is the level of complexity: can it vary or should there be standards?

- How do you disassociate from Environmental Impact Assessment "baggage"?

- Where will it be applied (e.g., the federal vs. the local level)?

- What is the role for incentives and training?

Additionally, workshop participants were asked to offer their ideas for initiatives that CDC could undertake that would help establish a practice of considering health impact when making land use, transportation planning, and other community design decisions. To follow are the general themes coming out of that discussion:

- Establish a sense of public health urgency for healthy community design

- Become a part of the DOT/EPA/HUD Partnership for Sustainable Communities

- Create incentive programs

- Encourage interdisciplinary involvement to ensure that health impact is considered in all projects and policies that affect the built environment

- Conduct HIAs on high profile projects to achieve outcomes in the built environment that improve public health

- Conduct and fund research to establish an evidence base that describes the relationship between health and the design of the built environment, one that can be used to guide built environment projects and policies

CDC then asked participants to consider what the professional groups they represent could do to support the healthy community design agenda. While many specific ideas were shared and are being pursued, here are the general concepts considered:

- Garner exposure for Healthy Community Design in industry presentations and publications

- Contribute to policy efforts

- Include health impact in continuing education and licensure requirements

- Promote to audiences who develop or retrofit neighborhoods the LEED for Neighborhood Development (LEED-ND) rating system and the STAR Community Index (being developed through a partnership among ICLEI-Local Governments for Sustainability, the U.S. Green Building Council, and the Center for American Progress).

All participants indicated a desire to continue the dialogue past the workshop through additional meetings and an online discussion forum.

Anyone interested in healthy community design can refer to the follow sources:

- CDC Healthy Community Design Website http://www.cdc.gov/healthyplaces

- Healthy Community Design News Listservhttp://www.cdc.gov/healthyplaces/listserv.htm

## II.    OVERVIEW

### a. Statement of purpose

After World War II, the built environment became characterized by large-scale construction and cost-efficient, homogeneous projects. Car ownership became widespread; land use became more sprawling as large-scale, high-capacity freeways began to dominate transportation infrastructure investment. Community design infrastructure became wide streets to accommodate more traffic, to the neglect of sidewalks, bike lanes, and useful public transit. Such an infrastructure deterred physical activity and the use of pollution-reducing alternate forms of transportation. The end result was widespread traffic congestion; increased commuting time; increased vehicle, pedestrian and biking crashes and injuries; a growing obesity epidemic; a rise in air pollution and respiratory illness; and a growing sense of disconnection between workplaces and homes.

Mounting scientific evidence suggests that community design characteristics can have an impact on a community's level of physical activity; respiratory and mental health; water quality; social equity; ability to age in place; and social capital. Interest in related initiatives, such as Leadership in Energy and Environmental Design (LEED) in building and neighborhood design, has migrated from fringe to center.

With all this in mind, CDC decided to hold a workshop that brought experts in the built environment together to collaborate, discuss, and debate.

## b. Meeting date, location, and agenda

On September 21 and 22, 2009, thought leaders in the built environment community convened at the Centers for Disease Control and Prevention (CDC) in Atlanta, Georgia to develop communication strategies for raising awareness about the health impact of community design decisions and its potential to save lives and healthcare dollars.

During the two-day workshop, attendees discussed the factors influencing their audiences' decision processes when considering the health impact of a project or policy, current notable healthy community design practices and policies, and the strengths and weaknesses of implementing tools like Health Impact Assessments (HIA). The group also discussed communication strategies for encouraging widespread adoption of industry best practices and policies that improve quality of life in the nation.

The desired outcome was for participants collaboratively to develop action steps to expand awareness of the health impact of community design decisions.

In 5–10 years, CDC hopes that the strategies developed from this workshop will lead to

- Increased public health awareness in their training among architects, planners, and transportation planners

- Recognition by public health professionals that collaborating with architects, planners, transportation planners, and developers is key to advancing healthy community design

- The promotion and publication of best practices by all relevant parties

- Consideration by all relevant parties of objectively evaluating the potential health effects of a project or policy before it is built or implemented.

## c. Attendees

Recognizing that collaboration among multiple sectors is critical to making healthy community design decisions a standard practice, CDC invited established experts—public health professionals, members of government agencies, planners, architects, academics, and developers—from across the country to participate in the panel. Organizations represented included the

- American Institute of Architects (AIA), Bill Gilchrist

- American Planning Association, Bill Klein

- American Society of Landscape Architects (ASLA), Paul Morris

- Congress for the New Urbanism, John Norquist

- Georgia Institute of Technology College of Architecture, Ellen Dunham-Jones

- International City/County Management Association, Amanda Thompson

- Local Government Commission, Judy Corbett

- McGuire Woods LLP, Daniel Slone

- National Association of County and City Health Officials, Jennifer Li

- National Association of Home Builders, Debra Bassert

- National Conference of State Legislatures, Doug Farquhar

- Health Impact Project (a collaboration of the Robert Wood Johnson Foundation and Pew Charitable Trusts), Aaron Wernham and Linda Paris

- Regional Plan Association, Robert Yaro

- Urban Land Institute, Art Lomenick

- U.S. Access Board, Peg Blechman

- U.S. Department of Housing and Urban Development, Ron Sims

- U.S. Environmental Protection Agency, Tim Torma

- U.S. Green Building Council, Susan Mudd

CDC invited representatives from the U.S. Department of Transportation, the American Association of State Highway and Transportation Officials, and the American Association of Retired Persons to participate in the event but none confirmed or attended.

## III.   WHAT IS HEALTHY COMMUNITY DESIGN?

### a. Summary of Andrew Dannenberg and Howard Frumkin's remarks

Dr. Andrew Dannenberg, Associate Director for Science, Division of Emergency and Environmental Health Services, National Center for Environmental Health (NCEH) at CDC and the team lead for CDC's Healthy Community Design Initiative, kicked off the event.  He spoke about the past eight years of the initiative's work in establishing a link between the built environment and health. Dannenberg stated that when he is asked the question, "What are you working on?" his short answer is, "When you want people to walk, you have to give them a place to walk." The longer answer is that community design impacts a number of health issues, including obesity, climate change, mental health, social equity, social capital, respiratory health, accessibility, and healthy aging.

Dannenberg addressed the importance of building and strengthening partnerships across many disciplines, and he pointed to some of the challenges.

"In some cases we don't even speak the same language," he said. "I was at a transportation meeting a few years ago and people kept saying NMT. How many of you know what NMT is? No one. It's non-motorized transportation. They meant biking and walking, but in the transportation world, they just kept saying NMT. There are other examples as we try to learn each other's language and how to move things forward."

He described the focus of the meeting as being more on communication and partnership building between health and the built environment than on science. "What are the messages, and how do we get a common vocabulary and work from that angle?"

Another key area of focus addressed by Dannenberg was how to reach decision-makers.

"Who are the people we need to reach? Most of them are outside the health field. We're talking about politicians, people working in transportation, in housing, and in other areas that are not primarily health areas. But, in fact, anyone working in those areas is impacting public health, and so as health people ourselves, we need to convey the message to people in these other fields that actually they're all part of the public health realm."

Dr. Howard Frumkin, who at that time was director of CDC's National Center for Environmental Health (NCEH) and the Agency for Toxic Substances and Disease Registry, also attended a portion of the event. He addressed four topics:

## 1) The importance of healthy community design

"We understand better and better from the CDC perspective that the major causes of morbidity and mortality in the country are profoundly affected by the issues of community design and built environment, so this is very much at the soul of what we do here."

## 2) The challenge regarding collecting evidence

"There is a culture difference between biomedical scientists and lots of the others at the table. We have the information in the health sciences in recent years to base everything we do on very solid ground. We like randomized clinical trials before we give you medications… We don't hold ourselves collectively to the same level of solid evidence when it comes to environmental design at NCEH. But we can make stronger cases for changes if we have good evidence, and if the evidence is thorough."

## 3) The benefits of collaboration

Using an example he gathered on a trip to Portland, Frumkin said, "There's a swale. It sits inside the curb… it's a small retention pond. This little piece of infrastructure is very effective as a way to protect bicycles from automobiles. It's also very good at managing storm water. The beauty of it is that it is half-funded by the water department and half-funded by the transportation department. It's a really nice example of how we get together and identify joint benefits that flow from single interventions and co-advocate and co-fund. We can get a lot more done than we ever could [by] working in our separate silos. It's going be the key to our success."

## 4) Culture changing

Frumkin referenced the article "The Green Case for Cities" by Witold Rybczynski in the October 2009 issue of *The Atlantic*. "The author's point is the environmental benefits of living in dense urban settings so far outweigh putting solar panels on your roof or doing other things in the suburbs because of the smaller space that you live in and the reduced energy demand of urban construction compared to Greenfield suburban construction. You reduce travel, and all of that has a much bigger environmental benefit than the little things that we do around the edges in the suburbs. The point is there's a profound set of advantages to changing people's orientation about the way they live, and his claim in this piece is more people need to, want to move to the cities. That means changing our preferences and that's culture change. We all need to learn to live with less space and use less energy. We need to learn to walk and bike more. These are behavior changes. They're culture changes. To the extent we achieve them, we'll achieve environmental gains and sustainability gains. We'll leave a better world to those who come after us. It's why communications in this meeting is so important, because ultimately what this is about is culture change. And it's only going to happen if we change culture, and that's only going to happen through effective communication which we carry out collaboratively based on strong evidence."

## IV.     WHO INFLUENCES HEALTHY COMMUNITY DESIGN/HOW DO THEY VIEW THE CURRENT SITUATION AND CDC'S ROLE?

### a. Summary of Jerry McCann's presentation

Jerry McCann, vice president and account leader for the marketing communications firm Carton Donofrio Partners, presented results from a series of interviews he conducted with built environment decision-makers. CDC retained Carton Donofrio Partners to develop a better understanding of influencers in the built environment and their attitudes toward public health factors. The interviews led to the creation of the expert workshop event.

To start, McCann spoke of Carton Donofrio Partners' history as a 40-year-old marketing communications firm in Baltimore. He addressed the firm's capabilities in the built environment and public health sectors and its philosophy, including its emphasis on research as a key underpinning informing all initiatives.

McCann recapped CDC's Healthy Community Design Initiative (HCDI) communication objectives:

- To increase awareness of public health factors related to the built environment among those who build and design communities

- To raise the priority on considering public health factors during the process of designing and renovating building communities and/or large-scale projects

Donofrio Partners' first step in achieving those goals was to gather the knowledge, attitudes and perceptions of HCDI's target audience through a series of open-ended interviews with members of the target audience. Among the interviewees were (1) a public health official from a major city, (2) a county planning commission member for a major metro area, (3) an American Institute of Architects member heavily involved in the rejuvenation of a riverfront in a major city, (4) a highly successful developer who is now a think-tank fellow, (5) a land use attorney employed by developers, (6) a district manager for a state department of transportation, and (7) a Federal Highway Administration official involved in bicycle and pedestrian projects. Conversation highlights are as follows:

- **The land use attorney** said there's no formal public health review process built into codes, processes, and protocols.

- **The state department of transportation district manager** said that in his language, public health means hazardous materials abatement, worker safety, and dust-dirt management during construction.

- **The county planning commissioner** said that when she began serving in 2006, the situation was that the planners were from Venus and the health officials were from Mars. She associates health impact assessments with landfill issues, Brownfield areas, and areas where semi-industrial facilities exist in proximity to residential areas.

- **The city planner** reported that her hunt for good data is very difficult. For example, she was trying to find a list of supermarkets in disadvantaged areas of the city and expected to find it at a licensing bureau. Months later, she finally found it at the health department. When she got there, the health department had no idea of the significance of its data to community design. The city planning and the health departments are in the same building on the same floor.

- **The architect** noted that when he hears about public health issues, he hears about features. Those developing senior living facilities, for example, have expectations of a campus-like approach. Neighborhood groups express public health issues as a need for playgrounds, and the economically disadvantaged are looking for intact sidewalks, street lighting, access to retail on foot, and well located public transit, all of which they see as features. He saw none of these features as relating to public health.

- **The developer** noted that for a large downtown turnaround project, the city would typically outsource a bid for a master plan with the developers and/or design firms. Other commercial interests would join in. "Health players are noticeably not included in these discussions and they should be."

- **The federal biking coordinator** said walking and biking advocates search him out. He also hears from local government people who are not familiar with the federal process. He served as a resource to university researchers. He occasionally hears from architects and seldom from developers. Local public health officials tend not to be among those who call him looking for information.

Two key themes emerged from the conversations:

- Common concern about health exists; common language less so.

- Almost no cross-discipline synergy exists on shared health concerns; local public health professionals are not in the loop at the critical early stages of project or policy planning.

All interviewees agreed that CDC, as one of the leading national authorities on public health issues, has the credibility to convene the conversation on these issues, and they would all welcome some leadership from the CDC. Carton Donofrio Partners recommended that CDC convene an expert panel to start the conversation among built environment thought leaders of all disciplines hosted by CDC.

He noted that all attendees were recruited through their professional associations to ensure that the best thought leaders were selected. Finally, he said that his firm would work to find the commonalities (i.e., shared goals) among the various disciplines in order to develop an action plan from the meeting.

## V.    WHERE IS HEALTHY COMMUNITY DESIGN WORKING?

### a. Best practice examples: summarize top five initiatives selected for group exercise

The group focused on specific examples of how healthy community design is working. Five of these examples became the key focus of an exercise in enhancing communication about successes. The five selected were:

- **Miami-Dade, Florida**

  Bill Gilchrist, a senior associate at EDAW/AECOM and an American Institute of Architects (AIA) member, briefed the group on his work with Miami-Dade County.

  He said the interesting thing about this case—which is an amendment to the comprehensive plan for Miami-Dade County that is related to urban design and aesthetics—is that government genuinely does want to link the community design component to indications of improved health within the community. Bill noted, "They're looking at it not only in terms of adopting regulations that relate specifically to improved health, but also to link physical design with aesthetic outcome."

  The Miami-Dade case involves tying the aspects of community health and improved neighborhoods with centralized commercial districts in those neighborhoods to indicate that when the environment is healthier, there is a more stable and more thriving economic community as well. Gilchrist referenced the University of Wisconsin-Madison's Center for Community Economic Development(http://www.uwex.edu/ces/cced/downtowns/index.cfm; the Maine Development Foundation's "Indicators of Livable Communities" (http://www.maine.gov/spo/boards/landandwater/reports/Indicators%20of%20Livable%20Communities.pdf) and" The Economic Benefit of a Walkable Community" (http://www.uwex.edu/ces/CCED/downtowns/ltb/lets/0703ltb.pdf) ; and a series of fact sheets prepared by the Local Government Commission that focus on livable communities

(http://www.lgc.org/issues/communitydesign/street_design.html).

- **Garland, Texas**

  Art Lomenick, managing director of developer Trammell Crow, referred to Garland, Texas as the premier example of a city that had every tool in place. He explained that Garland is located outside of Dallas with a population of 230,000 people. Trammel Crow put a mixed-use development project together for the town, tapping the progressive tools the government assembled. Most interestingly, the city restructured itself around the initiative. Additionally, the city engaged in several "discovery" activities that are usually assigned to the developer/designers, either as part of a pitch process or as the first assignment after winning on the basis of being chosen on qualifications alone. The city itself was in a better position to gather and interpret the data (e.g., on storm water capacity, power line placement, street grid planning, economic viability of different building types, etc.) and gave itself more time to do it than is normally given a developer. The quality of the data was higher as a result, and the acceptance of the data throughout the city team was better. The developer was able to begin on a more solid footing and did not have to "sell" the data to the city; it was already "presold." The developer was able to begin more quickly, and it completed a project that normally takes five years in nine months.

- **The Belmar Project in Lakewood, Colorado**

  Ellen Dunham-Jones, associate professor with the Georgia Institute of Technology's College of Architecture, described Belmar, a former 100-acre auto-dependent "dead mall" outside of Denver in Lakewood, Colorado. It is now about two-thirds built out as a pedestrian-centered residential and retail development with 22 urban blocks, walkable public streets, public and civic spaces, eight bus lines, a mix of housing types and price points, in mostly two- to four-story buildings built to very green standards, with both solar and wind energy generation built-in. Density was tripled on the site without adding another street signal.

She spoke about how all of the suburban retrofit examples in her book *Retrofitting Surburbia*—including Belmar—contribute to health in a variety of ways:

- Redirecting growth to existing infrastructure instead of to greenfield sites at the edges
- Reducing auto dependency and reaping multiple health impacts with that reduction: increased walkability, increased social capital and connectedness, increased density and transit, and decreased costs and contributions to air pollution.
- Regreening greyfield sites currently covered with asphalt—by daylighting culverted streams and increasing permeable surface with "town greens" and tree-lined streets.

Dunham-Jones also spoke of changing suburban demographics as a big driver for these projects—the increasing number of suburban households without children is fueling demand for more urban housing types and lifestyles in suburban locations, and this is reviving the tax base of leap-frogged communities. Most of the examples in her book happened through opportunism more than by plan.

"They were mostly market-driven in one way or another, but they had to overcome a lot of obstacles. As far as I know, public health was never at the table during the negotiations. There's a huge market demand for retrofitting—and a public demand as communities look for ways to redevelop the accelerating number of underperforming retail properties in the suburbs in particular, a lot of aging stuff."

Dunham-Jones expressed excitement about getting health engaged with urban design and development because the legal basis of our codes is the protection of health, safety, and welfare.

"For me, it's not just about getting the health officials at the table in terms of local decision-making. That's obviously very important, but we need to fundamentally build on that legal basis of protecting health, safety, and welfare and figure out how we get to the point of having Surgeon General warnings on zoning codes and subdivision regulations. Imagine the impact of, 'The Surgeon General warns: This zoning code may be bad for your community's health,' and really change the system."

- **Tysons Corner, Virginia**

  Paul Morris, executive vice president of Parsons Brinckerhoff and past president of the American Society of Landscape Architects (ASLA), spoke as ASLA's representative at the workshop. He briefed the group on Tysons Corner, which *USA Today* called "the most highly celebrated recent urban redevelopment project in the country." He said it was motivated by the economic opportunity associated with the extension of Washington, D.C.'s Metro rail line to Dulles International Airport. Underlying that was the realization that economic and demographic changes that needed to be addressed to retrofit what in the 1960s was considered one of the most innovative developments in the country.

The project transforms a textbook case of suburban sprawl into a true 21st century urban center that addresses the challenges of sustainable growth, energy conservation, environmental protection, affordable housing, and safe communities. "It has one of the most extraordinary transportation systems surrounding it, but you can't get into the development, "stated Morris. "And with an employment population rivaling that of downtown Washington, DC, it is scalable. It has the potential to become a community of 80,000 people. It illustrates that projects at a scalable level are those that actually have the capacity to bring into and put in place the missing infrastructure and armature that makes it possible to introduce more complex land use and transportation systems that are financially viable and support the environmental and social agendas that we're trying to advance more broadly."

- **Decatur, Georgia**

Amanda Thompson, Planning Director for the City of Decatur, Georgia and the International City/County Management Association representative at the workshop, told the group about her experience in conducting a rapid health impact assessment on Decatur's community transportation plan.

"It was the first place in the nation to look at that. The plan was done in the framework of active living, which means you have the opportunity to exercise every day as part of your daily life, which naturally requires complete streets because you're not getting exercise when you're driving."

She spoke about how Decatur changed its recreation department into an active living division specifically to focus on policy and programming to promote active living throughout all operations.

"Decatur is 4.2 square miles. Adjacent DeVry University is a greyfield site, 21 acres that chose to annex into the City of Decatur. Even though the annexation would mean a property tax increase, DeVry chose to annex because of Decatur's mixed-use zoning ordinance. We had the regulations in place that would enable DeVry to build what it wanted. So this wasn't tax abatement, it wasn't incentives. We had the right regulations in place that made DeVry want to be a part of our city."

At the end of her presentation, Thompson asked, "Who benefits in everything that I'm working and looking at? And that's a fundamental health question. Who benefits, and are we being transparent about what's happening?"

## VI.    WHAT STEPS DO WE NEED TO TAKE TO ENCOURAGE WIDESPREAD ADOPTION OF INDUSTRY BEST PRACTICES?

a.  **Core ideas coming out of Communications breakout groups**

Following are the key action-oriented steps that surfaced from the Communications breakout groups. Items are broken into common themes: research, leadership/ownership, messaging/communications/marketing, financials, and strategy.

**RESEARCH**

Lack of hard, evidence-based health research was a challenge in every case study discussed. Suggestions for solutions included the following:

- **Use what we have now: powerful anecdotes and testimonials.**

  One participant noted, "It's going be a long time before we get performance measures. What we can use right now are the testimonials."

- **Develop a National Academy of the Built Environment**

  "We have the National Science Foundation, the National Academy of Science… none focuses on the built environment," a participant noted. "There's a case to be made that there should be direct Congressional funding for research on these issues. This is a place where CDC could make an impact."

- **Create a clearinghouse**

  One of the groups had a vision for a clearinghouse developed by CDC. "We talked about the clearinghouse as not only being a central place for data, best practices, and research, but also an area where people could talk about hurdles or stumbling blocks that exist because of local and federal government regulations."

- **Analyze**

  At Tysons Corner, the city "developed a new model called CFIT, which is a GIS-based analytical program. It creates a carbon footprint analysis that shows per capita carbon impact based on existing proposed alternative scenarios; it is now being exported to the State of California to use as a tool by federally-mandated and federally-funded metropolitan planning organizations to model their compliance with AB 32 [a law to reduce and eventually cap statewide emissions of greenhouse gases] and SB 375 [a law to reduce greenhouse gas emissions by curbing sprawl]."

- **Spotlight smaller markets doing it right**

  Several participants noted that the second- and third-tier outer ring suburban communities are making the fastest progress in achieving viable healthy community designs, and the accomplishments of these communities should be highlighted.

**LEADERSHIP/OWNERSHIP**

Not surprisingly, leadership was critical in each case discussed. Recommendations around this issue include the following:

- **Identify a champion**

  All the successful projects had a champion associated with them—in Tysons Corner and Garland, for example, it was the county commission board members. A willing leader or a group of leaders able to shepherd new plans, policies, and organizational structures through is a key ingredient to success.

- **Engage a broad constituency**

  Multiple participants said that grassroots or neighborhood participation in the process drove a sense of ownership and was a key to success.

- **Establish tag teams**

  Everyone agreed on the potential positive impact that health organizations and persons focused on health could make on the projects. One participant noted "The CDC—and many health organizations at the local and state levels—really have a potentially significant role to play in helping to define the parameters and standards by which we create and identify what a healthy community is and do it in a way that actually establishes a platform for using health terminology as a basis for defining successful communities."

  However, Paul Morris noted that most of the projects do not have health professionals at the table. Regarding Tysons Corner, a participant said, "This [project] was all driven by investment and fear. The project was an economic patient. It was not an environmental patient. I don't think I ever heard 'healthy communities' in any of the conversations."

  Another participant suggested tag teams: "The design professional would accompany the health professional and start getting the word out about how critically linked these aspects of the professions are for its healthy outcomes in community design." He went on to say, "If you're talking to the health community, you need a health professional with you to talk their language. If you're talking to the fire marshals, you need a fire person with you."

## MESSAGING, COMMUNICATIONS, and MARKETING

The right approach to messaging and marketing proved critical in all of the cases discussed.

- **Characterize healthy communities from an economic perspective**

  Several participants stressed the importance of promoting the economic benefits that come from creating more healthy communities.

- **Marketing health matters when communities don't really know what they want**

  Ellen Dunham-Jones said that in Belmar's case, the community originally wanted the dead mall to be revived. As a suburb, the community did not want or feel they particularly needed a "downtown." However, the lack of options and the degree to which the retrofit was presented as "green" changed attitudes, and the town has now fully embraced it. Additionally, Belmar's tagline, "Enrich your life; not your lawn," resonated well with both the young professionals and the retiring boomers.

- **Tell the lemons-to-lemonade story**

  Dunham-Jones advocated putting the focus on what people will gain from living in sustainable communities. "The media tends to focus on bad news and so much of the messaging on sustainability has been about how we have to sacrifice more. If we can demonstrate that living in more sustainable communities brings more happiness, we'll have a very powerful message."

- **Get the message out beyond those who already "get it"**

  Paul Morris stated "I don't think we should presume because we "get it" at the conceptual scale that the majority of organizations and groups out there or elected officials, planning commissions, city councils, county managers, or citizens at large do." Other participants suggested communications tactics such as a speakers' bureau and outreach to faith-based organizations.

- **Find terms that resonate**

  Amanda Thompson said that for the City of Decatur, the term *active living* helped move the city toward bike- and pedestrian-friendly roadways.

- **Focus the discussion on health**

  Thompson also said that the City of Decatur convened community members for an HIA. Looking at the project from a health perspective with community members helped focus the discussion and avoid its derailment.

- **Fish where the fish are**

  One participant emphasized the need to use new media for message dissemination such as podcasts, YouTube videos and Facebook fan pages."

**FINANCIALS**

- **Rethink the tax base**

  A participant noted that the tax base for municipalities is focused on retail, and this explains why many places are over-zoned for retail development. "We have about seven times as much retail in shopping centers as Europeans; almost double Australia and Canada."

- **Identify funding sources**

  In the Garland, Texas case, the city put in money first before the developer came along. Garland invested in removing the roadblocks first. The group discussed the idea of CDC grant money that would be tied to eligible activities, including those that would increase usage of public transit and non-motorized transportation, such as biking and walking.

- **Successes need to be created, not just catalogued**

  One participant suggested that HUD "should be providing some very modest incentive funding for demonstration projects, not just catalog the successes but create the successes."

**STRATEGY**

- **Make sure the community is mixed-use**

  Morris acknowledged that in many communities, creating more healthy communities that are mixed-use is actually illegal due to zoning laws. Tysons

Corner prohibited residential housing initially. Then, when the team re-imagined it, the city decided not only to permit residential but to allow it anywhere. The city added a 20 percent bonus to any project that provided residential construction. The city understood that there was an inextricable link between the number of jobs available in Tysons Corner and the amount of residential housing that could be supported by it. The city knew that to create a vibrant, healthy community, it had to create a place for people to live where they worked.

- **Aim for strategic scalability**

  In discussing retrofitting dead malls, Dunham-Jones stressed the importance of looking at all the potential re-developable properties within a municipality, within a metro region, and then planning strategically. Which ones get redeveloped so that density is increased and transit makes sense? Which do you try to re-green because they are a part of some natural system corridor?

- **Consider the demographics**

  Several different cases addressed the issue of demographics associated with aging, young urban, and immigrant populations. Morris noted, "We're still building about 85 percent of our housing in the suburban single-family model for the traditional 'nuclear family', even though all projections show that up to 70 percent will be one- and two-person households, and at least 50 percent of future housing demand will be for non-single families. We don't have a homebuilding industry that's prepared for that kind of market transformation, so we have to reorganize around this new paradigm to make success possible." Another participant made a related point: "We need to be tapping into these audiences, both in terms of a better understanding of how design impacts their concerns but also finding out how they can inform us to be more effective in our outreach and implementation of design and of legal adoption of ordinances, comprehensive plan elements, regulations, overlays, etc."

## VII. TOOL FOR EVALUATING OBJECTIVELY THE POTENTIAL HEALTH EFFECTS OF A PROJECT OR POLICY BEFORE IT IS BUILT OR IMPLEMENTED: HEALTH IMPACT ASSESSMENT (HIA)

Dannenberg provided an overview of the Health Impact Assessment (HIA), followed by a discussion among all participants about the opportunities and challenges associated with its implementation.

### a. Definition

HIA is a collection of procedures and tools for which projects, policies, and programs can be evaluated based on their potential effects on the health of the population, particularly health disparity issues.

HIA is one of the tools available to facilitate communication and partnerships among health professionals, designers, architects, and other decision-makers on the built environment.

The vision for HIA:

- Planners and others will request information on potential health consequences of projects and policies as part of their decision-making process

- Health officials will have a tool to facilitate their involvement in planning and land use decisions

- HIAs will lead to better informed decisions

An HIA has six basic steps:

1. Screening: Which projects/policies could benefit?

2. Scoping: Which health impacts should be looked at?

3. Risk Assessment: How will people be affected? How many?

4. Recommendation: What can be done about it?

5. Reporting: How do we get the information to the decision-makers?

6. Evaluation: What is the effect on the decision process?

HIA gives health a "voice" at the table when planning and land use decisions are being made.

## b. State of the HIA

Frequency of Use

HIAs are more prevalent in Europe than in the United States, according to John Kemm, West Midlands Public Health Observatory, United Kingdom. CDC's Healthy

Community Design Initiative found that, at the end of 2008, approximately 39 HIAs had been completed in the United States. As of mid-2009, this number had grown to around 60. Completed HIAs can be difficult to track; more HIAs may exist of which CDC is unaware.

## Voluntary vs. Regulatory

Much of the discussion around HIAs today is about whether they should be voluntary or regulatory. According to Dannenberg, "If a health official voluntarily uses them to convey health information to a planning agency, the process is simpler, less expensive, and less litigious."

The drawback is that a voluntary HIA is less likely to be used. On the other hand, a regulatory model or an environmental impact statement is more complex, expensive, and litigious. Health impact can actually fit within the scope of an environmental impact statement. The latter is not needed for all projects and policies; in some instances, an HIA should be considered separately.

## Quantitative vs. Qualitative

Much talk exists about whether a HIA should be measured qualitatively or quantitatively. Providing directional health impacts is relatively easy (e.g., if you build more sidewalks, people will have more access to physical activity). While some quantitative data are available, proving health benefits with numbers requires complex modeling that does not readily exist today.

## Effectiveness

Looking back after a project or policy is implemented and determining whether an HIA made a difference is ideal. Some impacts, such as pedestrian safety, adoption of living wage ordinances, and access to replacement housing, have been documented. The other measure of effectiveness is whether an HIA raised awareness of the decision-makers and influenced their behavior. Another key component of effectiveness is the level of community involvement.

## Health Impact Project (a collaboration of the Robert Wood Johnson Foundation and Pew Charitable Trusts)

The Robert Wood Johnson Foundation (RWJF) and the Pew Charitable Trusts (Pew) launched the Health Impact Project, a national initiative designed to promote the use of HIAs as a decision-making tool for policymakers.  Dr. Aaron Wernham, director of the Health Impact Project, presented background on the initiative. As a practicing physician, Wernham noticed that the prevalence of diabetes among his patients increased from 5 to more than 50 percent in just 10 years. He touched on the phenomenal wave of chronic disease in the United States and how it can be linked directly and indirectly to environmental issues, including the built environment. He reminded the group that not all health decisions are made within a doctor's office or even within a public health system. His position is that while we understand the problems, few tools exist to address them. RWJF has been funding a modest number of HIA projects in the United States that yielded promising results. This led to the funding of a center at Pew to test and demonstrate the efficacy of the HIA. The Health Impact Project will provide grants to fund HIAs, as well as training and technical assistance to grantees. The aim of the Health Impact Project is to promote effective strategies for supporting and institutionalizing the use of HIAs.

## c. Real and perceived barriers

Participants were given the opportunity to comment on the challenges and opportunities of HIAs. The following questions were posed:

<u>What should be the level of complexity for HIA: can it vary or should there be standards?</u>

"…in terms of dealing with developers, the last thing they'd ever want would be more process…. if you put in another layer and you have to hire a health impact assessment consultant, it's going to put [the developer] out of business, and he actually wants to do the right thing."

"…should HIA be at different levels from the highly complex [the projects and policies] down to the simple? …I think you need a whole range of HIAs, depending on complexity, time and resources."

<u>How do you disassociate HIA from Environmental Impact Assessment (EIA) baggage (e.g., National Environmental Policy Act which is designed to stop negative environmental impact vs. encouraging better health outcomes; not just barriers, but disincentives because EIAs increase time and cost)?</u>

"… industry is adopting health impact assessment as part of the project planning if there is a business case that can be made for it—addressing issues head-on and early in your project design and planning rather than waiting for the litigation that can potentially develop later. So I do think the concerns about NEPA are valid, and I do not think it's the ideal vehicle for most health impact assessment…but I think it's important to recognize that it's not necessarily going to slow everything down if you do one."

"There are many NEPAs in different states that are not as disruptive as the national NEPA is. They are potential plug-in points where there's a balancing process when we look at these things."

Where should HIA be applied (e.g., federal vs. local level; part of planning vs. "rear-guard" action in the regulatory process)?

"…if HIA ends up down at the deal-by-deal level, it's a showstopper."

"The comprehensive plan is where public health input is critical and is not addressed …but then the next big question would be are we going to make compliance with the comprehensive plan mandatory…?"

"I think a great legal access point would be at the code creation point and making sure that all of the aspects of human health were being addressed. I agree with the voluntary component [of HIA], but the percentage of impact on a voluntary component is relatively low still…"

"I think you would be far better off if you went to the front end in planning and built it into the process that sets the stage for all development later and built in certainty for developers to know, what the rules of the game are in particular areas. Then you're not going to get bogged down into the kind of bickering that occurs, and you'll come out with something that makes better sense, instead of being project-by-project, to get more of a systematic approach."

## What is the role for incentives and training?

"These programs [e.g., U.S. Green Building Council's LEED-ND] are designed to create voluntary systematic approaches to give incentives and instruction on how to do the right [health and built environment] thing and to create rewards and mechanisms for people to do it well so that they're not relying on their own institutional memory and some political jurisdiction that doesn't fully know the story."

"…making HIA available as a training regimen…for public health officials to become more active participants in this conversation at the local level would be extraordinarily powerful…I don't know any of them personally who actually participate in community planning and development discussions, let alone decisions…for every public health department or agency to have an advocate who is knowledgeable on HIA to participate in the process, I think that has the potential to contribute to some transformative change."

"…there are all these great think tanks and conferences that go on. Well, guess who never gets to go? It's municipal people because they won't spend the money. So you end up with a bunch of architects and planners and lawyers and economic development people…"

"…the accreditation standards for each discipline are certainly one of the ways in which areas do get brought in to all of the different disciplines…almost all of our professions require continuing education; that's an opportunity on the education side."

"…[HIA] could be a great set of criteria for establishing grants or incentive programs to promote demonstration projects because what you're creating through this is a series of indicators that could serve as principles for effective and healthy communities, and if this becomes part of that mechanism to institute it, you're going to see prospective applicants coming forward…"

## VIII.  THE PATH FORWARD

Following is a series of ideas for what CDC and participating industry groups can do to forward the mission. For specific action items from the meeting, please see "**b. Keeping the conversation going**" at the end of this report.

### a. Summarize ideas for CDC initiatives

Workshop participants were asked to offer their ideas for initiatives CDC could undertake that would help establish a practice of considering health impact when making land use, transportation planning, and other community design decisions.

## Establish a Sense of Urgency for Healthy Community Design

Participants provided several examples of public health crises that led to positive behavior change and recommended that CDC consider how to provide the same sense of urgency to healthy community design. Some caution was expressed about the public's suffering from crisis fatigue and, to that end, the need to ensure that any messaging not conflict with what other programs at CDC are saying.

"Say to yourselves, 'Healthy communities are a crisis and we have institutions within CDC for how we treat these crises, and how would we apply that…process to this question?'…you would clearly be elevating it to a level of importance that it is not [at] right now…and you would be taking advantage of methodologies and practices that are already systematic within the CDC organization and using them in a different way."

"We're talking about a wave of chronic disease, a tidal wave really—asthma and diabetes, obesity, and related conditions…would there be a way to make a more functional sort of partnership between the National Center for Chronic Disease and the National Center for Environmental Health?"

"...a lot of the burden of disease in the U.S. is related to the [decisions] that planners and transportation officials and businesses are [making] ... CDC needs to think, 'How do we restructure...to respond to a public health threat, which is being generated across multiple sectors that don't interact much with public health?'"

"...because of the chronic diseases...tens of millions of Americans are going to die earlier, [and there will be] colossal impacts on the economy and on the public health system and the cost of healthcare."

"...focusing on both the health impact on kids and I would try to go beyond toxins and obesity issues...I really do think [we should focus on] mental health, the levels of depression and suicide amongst non-drivers in suburbia."

"I think the most important thing I can say is that we have a conversation going on in this country about the health system and what better time to talk about our concern about the built environment and talking about how the built environment is the single most important preventive measure that we have at our disposal over the long term?"

Enter DOT/EPA/HUD Partnership

Participants learned about a new partnership for sustainable communities that includes the U.S. Department of Transportation (DOT), the U.S. Environmental Protection Agency (EPA), and the U.S. Department of Housing and Urban Development (HUD). It is designed to help improve access to affordable housing, increase transportation options, and lower transportation costs while protecting the environment in communities nationwide. Participants felt strongly that CDC (or its parent, the Department of Health and Human Services) should be included.

"I think CDC should look at other federal agencies, enter this partnership that HUD, DOT, and EPA started, and look for standards that [HUD, EPA and DOT] currently use that encourage sprawl and unhealthy living."

"I am eager about looking at how we can integrate CDC into the HUD and EPA and DOT [partnership]…I think there's an opportunity here to build some alliances and get these considerations right in the heart of this new approach the federal government is going to be taking to housing and urban policy and transportation."

Create Incentive Programs

Participants suggested that local jurisdictions would be more responsive to considering health impact if there were specific incentives to do so.

"I think we can do it with some modest incentives [like U.S. Department of Transportation's Safety Incentive Grants for Use of Seat Belts: http://www.nhtsa.dot.gov/nhtsa/whatsup/tea21/GrantMan/HTML/19b_Sec157InctReg 23CFR1240.html]. Again, if you can get every state to adopt a seatbelt law with 1 percent [incentive], you can get every state to adopt new street design [requirements] for 1 percent, and I think we ought to focus on some easy targets like that."

Provide Data and Success Stories

Participants felt there are not enough hard data to encourage decision-makers about the benefits of healthy community design. They also wanted to see quantifiable success stories.

"…CDC could look at research that has to do with road metrics and zoning and mixed use zoning issues…if you understood the issues and then weighed in, particularly talking to other agencies…you can speak with authority, and I think that would be a big help."

"…if you are able to take…information directly linking pedestrianism and health, we can support form-based codes…we can plant that in every legislative discussion that goes forward on a form-based code, whether it's SmartCode or otherwise."

"…there has been inadequate analysis to show that [communities designed for active living] are successful at what we hold them out to accomplish…show me that has happened…."

Encourage Interdisciplinary Involvement

Participants suggested that the only way to effect real change would be to foster collaboration among groups that are not used to working together. They felt the workshop was an important demonstration of this point. Another imperative was to ensure public health professionals have a voice in how built environment decisions are made. Three of the challenges presented were the need for a common nomenclature, a concerted training effort, and a better understanding of the process to predict where there may be friction. There were also several comments about incorporating healthy community design into academic curricula.

"…It's not just about professionals out there, whether they be city managers or planners. It's also the elected officials."

"The role I would love to see local public health officials play is that they become partners—they join up with…local chapters of APA [American Planning Association], CNU [Congress for the New Urbanism], ULI [Urban Land Institute], all the various organizations…who want to apply for incentives…and their role is to help talk to the elected officials and say, 'Look opportunities [to improve public health] are out there..'"

"…I've worked with public health agencies who…when you bring up the question about healthy communities, they think that's somebody else's job …'"

"…you need to get the health official on the panel, [but] they also need to be qualified to actually perform and conduct some help in that panel, and I've seen health professionals put on panels…who didn't know what to do to contribute."

"Things I've learned here [at the workshop]…should be brought…to environmental organizations to urge their involvement in these issues at the local level."

Conduct HIAs on High Profile Projects

Participants thought inclusion of an HIA in projects that are garnering attention would be an effective way to demonstrate their importance and benefits.

"I want to talk…about the idea of adding a health impact assessment [to the Times Square pedestrianization project] to see if we can calculate the health benefits… There are tens of millions of people who now have had an extra walk or an extra day of being a pedestrian instead of driving in Manhattan…I think this can play the same kind of role that the New York City smoking ban did [in improving public health]…"

**b. The contributions that industry groups can make**

CDC asked participants to consider what the professional groups they represent could do to support the healthy community design agenda. While many specific ideas were shared and are being pursued (see "**b. Keeping the conversation going**" at the end of this report), the following is a summary of the general concepts.

Garner Exposure in Industry Presentations and Publications

Several participants offered industry conference presentations and/or Webinars as a means of spreading the word on healthy community design among their peers. Specific suggestions included keynote speeches, committee presentations, and co-sponsored Webcasts. Additionally, a number of participants felt exposure in their association-sponsored publications would help reach others in their profession. Specific ideas included sponsored content, dedicated issues, bylined articles, and co-published thought pieces (e.g., Ten Principles of Healthy Community Design with ULI).

Contribute to Policy Efforts

Virtually every participant talked about his or her organization's policy-related initiatives. While CDC cannot lobby, participants felt that CDC could have a voice in the organizations' efforts to educate lawmakers. Several specific opportunities were shared, including participation in Livable Communities legislation and involvement in America 2050 (a national initiative to meet the infrastructure, economic development, and environmental challenges of the nation, http://www.america2050.org/).

Additionally, one of the barriers to healthy community design is that some existing transport laws do not allow communities to build complete streets. Several attendees spoke about the importance of changing legislation on this issue, and many said this portion of the conversation would have been more productive had a transportation person attended. As mentioned, transportation representatives were invited but did not respond.

Include Health Impact in Continuing Education and Licensure Requirements

Many professional organizations represented require their members to earn continuing education credits to maintain their licensure. Participants felt that CDC could contribute content to continuing education programs for these organizations. Participants whose professions require licensure felt that their organizations' licensure programs could incorporate health impact requirements. Next-generation professionals would be tested and granted a license partly on the basis of their understanding of and commitment to upholding healthy community design principles.

One participant who volunteers for the U.S. Green Building Council's LEED for Neighborhood Development (LEED-ND, http://www.usgbc.org/DisplayPage.aspx?CMSPageID=148) suggested that there may be a way to incorporate health impact into LEED-ND as an innovation credit. The first version of LEED-ND was recently finalized, and projects can be submitted in 2010. While it is too late for health impact to be incorporated in the first rating system, it was suggested that it may be considered for the future iterations. There will be a core committee responsible for the rewrite, and the participants encouraged someone from CDC to pursue inclusion.

## IX.    CONCLUSION

### a. Summarize participant evaluations

Expert panel participants were asked to complete a brief evaluation form following the workshop. Findings overall suggested that participants viewed the workshop very positively. The opportunity to meet other participants was overwhelmingly cited as the most valuable component. They also expressed interest in participating in additional workshops on this topic and in joining an online community to continue the discussion that was started at the event.

Participants were asked to discuss the barriers to and opportunities for moving the health agenda forward among built environment decision-makers. Findings indicated that respondents were much more likely to discuss and elaborate on perceived barriers rather than opportunities. Challenges that were frequently mentioned included the complexity of issues and relationships, the lack of a sense of urgency, funding shortfalls, and the lack of message clarity. Strategies to increase the health agenda included having data to support goals and building local and community knowledge.

Participants were asked to provide strategies for CDC to help move the health agenda forward. Suggestions included strengthening old partnerships and developing new partnerships, as well as actively promoting the link between health and the built environment.

## b. Keeping the conversation going

Several communications channels are available to people who are interested in healthy community design and the continued discussion from the Healthy Community Design Expert Workshop. They are as follows:

- CDC Healthy Community Design Website http://www.cdc.gov/healthyplaces
- Healthy Community Design News Listserv
  http://www.cdc.gov/healthyplaces/listserv.htm

Meeting participants offered the following opportunities for CDC's Healthy Community Design Initiative to work more closely with their organizations and affiliations:

- Robert Yaro, of the Regional Plan Association, suggested that PlaNYC (http://www.plannyc.org/) will do an economic assessment by the end of 2010 and will be adding health impact. Additionally, he's working on America 2050 and would like to explore the opportunity for CDC to have a voice in that program to ensure that public health factors are considered.

- Sharunda Buchanan, Director of the Division of Emergency and Environmental Health Services at CDC's National Center for Environmental Health, invited select outside stakeholders to participate in CDC Grand Rounds, as appropriate.

- Ellen Dunham-Jones of Georgia Institute of Technology's College of Architecture is creating a retrofitting suburbia class to which CDC could have input and provide a guest speaker.

- Paul Morris of American Society of Landscape Architects (ASLA) proposed multiple opportunities with ASLA communications. Additionally, he talked about the organization's partnerships with universities, its role on Capitol Hill, and the landscape architectural registration board.

- Amanda Thompson, representing International City/County Management Association (ICMA), suggested a CDC keynote speaking engagement at an upcoming ICMA event.

- Bill Klein, representing the American Planning Association (APA), mentioned that participants can find out more about APA's initiatives relating to the relationship between community design and health by visiting APA's Planning and Community Health Research Center at http://www.planning.org/nationalcenters/health/index.htm . He noted that its new online forum will be unveiled in early 2010.

- Doug Farquhar of the National Conference of State Legislatures (NCSL) proposed efforts in reaching his members through NCSL press releases, Webinars, and podcasts that highlight state activities that can be tied back to examples of CDC healthy community design guidelines in action. CDC advisors could also be called upon when legislators want to know more about health impact assessment. NCSL has also had success in creating videos on specific health-related topics as resources for legislators who want to know more about an issue or present it to others.

- Bill Gilchrist of American Institute of Architects (AIA) said AIA has internal committees such as the environment committee that he can invite CDC representatives to attend and speak at. Additionally, AIA gathers information on best practices to advance the conversation, and CDC could contribute to AIA's efforts. He also referenced the AIA convention as an opportunity for CDC's Healthy Community Design Initiative to gain exposure.

- Judy Corbett of the Local Government Commission (LGC) said that on February 4–6, 2010, LGC is hosting the New Partners for Smart Growth conference in Seattle, Washington. She welcomed CDC's help in public health training.

- Jennifer Li of National Association of County and City Health Officials (NACCHO) mentioned her organization's involvement with the ACHIEVE initiative and CDC's National Center for Chronic Disease Prevention and Health Promotion. She pointed to a co-sponsored Webcast focused on injury prevention, smart growth, and community design. She volunteered to work with ACHIEVE colleagues to spread the word through the ACHIEVE communities that are being funded. Additionally, she referenced an upcoming mentorship project on health impact assessment and talked about the NACCHO model practices program, which captures some of the success stories.

###